Exercise for Weight Loss

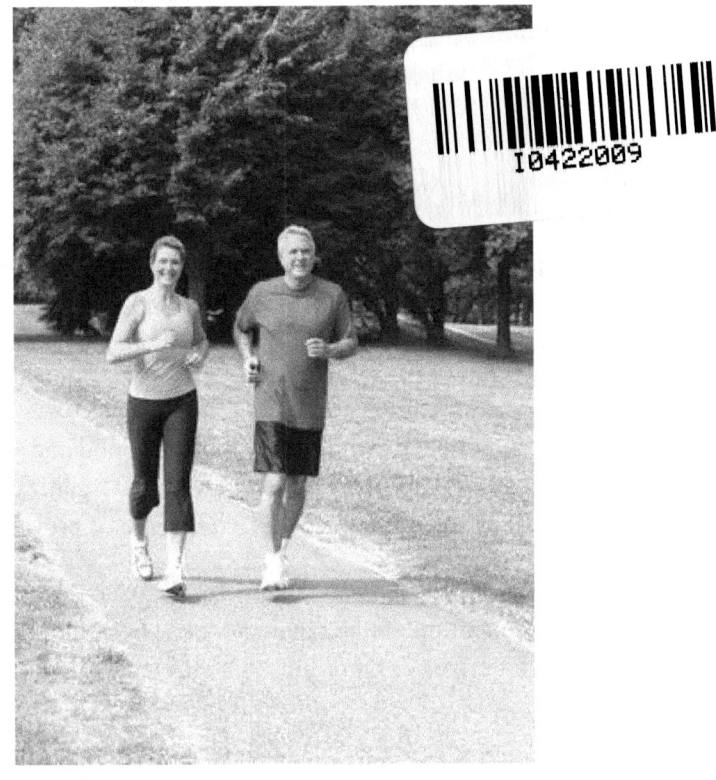

Health Learning Series

M. Usman

Mendon Cottage Books

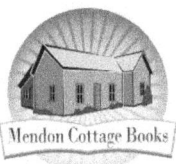

JD-Biz Publishing

Disclaimer

The information is this book is provided for informational purposes only. It is not intended to be used and medical advice or a substitute for proper medical treatment by a qualified health care provider. The information is believed to be accurate as presented based on research by the author.

The contents have not been evaluated by the U.S. Food and Drug Administration or any other Government or Health Organization and the contents in this book are not to be used to treat cure or prevent disease.

The author or publisher is not responsible for the use or safety of any diet, procedure or treatment mentioned in this book. The author or publisher is not responsible for errors or omissions that may exist.

Warning

The Book is for informational purposes only and before taking on any diet, treatment or medical procedure, it is recommended to consult with your primary health care provider.

Our books are available at
1. Amazon.com
2. Barnes and Noble
3. Itunes
4. Kobo
5. Smashwords
6. Google Play Books

Table of Contents

Preface..4

Getting Started 5

    Chapter # 1: Benefits of Exercise.................................5

    Chapter # 2: Exercise & Weight Loss.........................9

    Chapter # 3: Exercise & the Body..............................14

Hard-core Work Out 18

    Chapter # 1: Introduction 18

    Chapter # 2: Mondays 22

    Chapter # 3: Tuesdays and Thursdays.......................24

    Chapter # 4: Wednesdays...26

    Chapter # 5: Fridays 28

    Chapter # 6: Alternate 30

Conclusion 31

References..32

Author Bio...33

Publisher..44

Preface

Obesity is one of the biggest problems of our generation and the generations that follow. It is inflating at a rate that it can't be controlled and the only true way to control it is so hard that people tend to shift toward ways that provide them temporary relief but long-term problems. The most common types of temporary solutions are the take-the-pill solution and dieting, but the body can't come to terms with its original shape until and unless a person starts to exercise.

You know what exercise is; any activity that involves physical activity or work being done. Regular exercise is very important and not only necessary for losing weight but also for keeping it off. Exercise has been here, in our lives, since our inception and in one way or another we have been doing some kind of physical activity. But in today's ultra-fast world, physical activity has been reduced drastically and even going to a nearby grocery store is considered too much work. Thus, a person starts to gain weight, along with several other harmful conditions, and lose shape. This book is focused on exercise and will tell you the means as to how to lose weight through it.

But before you begin, it is advised that you check up with your doctor to see that you don't have a medical condition that may become more intensified as time goes on. If exercise is something you seldom do, then it is advised that you wait 21 days and get yourself ready for it; only then should you start up with a physical activity.

The book will take you through the benefits, the basics and types of exercises required to lose weight.

Getting Started

Chapter # 1: Benefits of Exercise

People spend more than half of their lives sitting, and that's the waking half. The other half is usually spent performing activities that don't do anything good for the body. This trend has been growing in the new generation and people are failing to realize this. Studies based on observation are suggesting that inactivity as a habit can raise the risk of diabetes, cardiovascular disease, obesity, and metabolic syndrome.

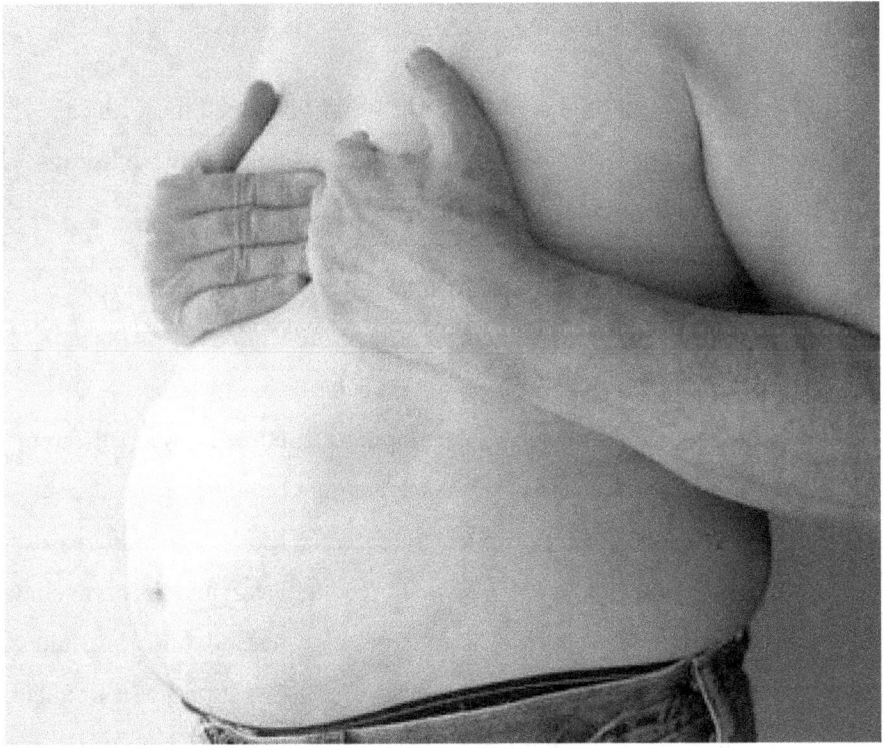

One study in fact, was able to show that middle aged women who seldom moved, watched TV, and were habitually inactive gained more weight and had a higher risk of developing diabetes; the study followed 50,000 middle aged females for almost 6 years. Every two hours that women spend watching TV, they add the risk of gaining weight by 23%. Moreover, they increased their risk of getting diabetes by 14%. Also, it was found out that individuals who spent most of their times sitting had increased risk of obesity. Therefore, when planning out the day it would be beneficial if you put some physical activity in it, as with the passage of time, inactivity will turn into a habit which will only have adverse effects on you.

The case for exercise is thus very strong, and decade's worth of solid science confirms that adding just as much as half an hour worth of exercise daily can improve your lifestyle.

Exercise packs in a lot of benefits, not just weight loss, and these all can become potential motivators for you. Therefore, a comprehensive list of benefits followed by a detailed chapter wise outlook is given.

1.   It lessens the chances of contracting heart disease which is the number 1 killer disease in the whole of the United States for both men and women. Exercising on a regular basis stops the accumulation of plaque by developing a fine line between different types of cholesterol, as well as triglycerides, and helps the arteries retain their resilience despite aging effects. Exercise also increases the number of blood vessels which feed the heart and thus prevent a heart attack. Moreover, it discourages clotting, inflammation, and arteries blocakage and lowers the chances of death from heart attack if you currently have it.

2.   It prevents diabetes by shaving off excessive weight, boosting sensitivity to insulin, and lowering levels of blood sugar. When

sensitivity to blood sugar is boosted, it results in less glucose being transported to cells, so if you have diabetes, the condition would get better.

3. Exercise lowers blood pressure which is a boon for many individuals. Long term high blood pressure or hypertension can double or even triple the chances of contracting heart disease, which paves the way for many other disease like aortic aneurysms, strokes, and kidney diseases.

4. Exercise also reduces the risk of developing cancers like colon and breast cancers; some studies even show it helps in preventing cancers of the uterine lining. It accomplishes this by helping you attain a healthy weight.

5. It helps make the bones strong. When bearing exercises like sprinting and walking or strength training is combined with vitamins like vitamin D, the result is bone protecting mechanisms which keeps diseases like osteoporosis away.

6. Exercise also protects the joints by easing up pain, fatigue, and swelling. It keeps the cartilage healthy and as the muscles start to develop, they lighten up the load on the joints.

7. By helping you control weight, it may reverse knee problems which would be the biggest bang for the buck. It is well known that every pound of weight lost reduces 4 pounds of weight over the knee.

8. Exercise also lifts one's mood by releasing hormones that relieve stress. Some studies have shown that individuals who exercise

regularly are able to counter their depression levels as efficiently as some medications.

9.   Exercise is known to add years to one's life. In the Framingham Heart Study, a moderate amount of activity increased a man's life by 1.3 years whereas it increased a women's life by 18 months. When the bar was raised much higher, men lived 3.7 years longer while women lived 3.5 years more.

Chapter # 2: Exercise & Weight Loss

What exactly goes on inside the body when you take a stroll or go for a swim? Any physical activity creates a complicated set of physical processes that have effects on almost every organ. Like all machines or moving entities, the muscles require and have fuel. The fuel comes from the food a person eats or the one that is stored in the body as a reserve in the form of either fat or glucose. The only loop is that the food cannot be directly converted into fuel ready to be burnt in the trillions of cells in the body. In fact, each cell has its own storage location for energy and the molecule stored in it is known as ATP or adenosine triphosphate. The body's ability to manufacture ATP is very vital as it determines the volume of physical exertion the muscles can bear. The vice versa is also true in this case, as the amount of muscle conditioning decides whether you can generate sufficient ATP or not.

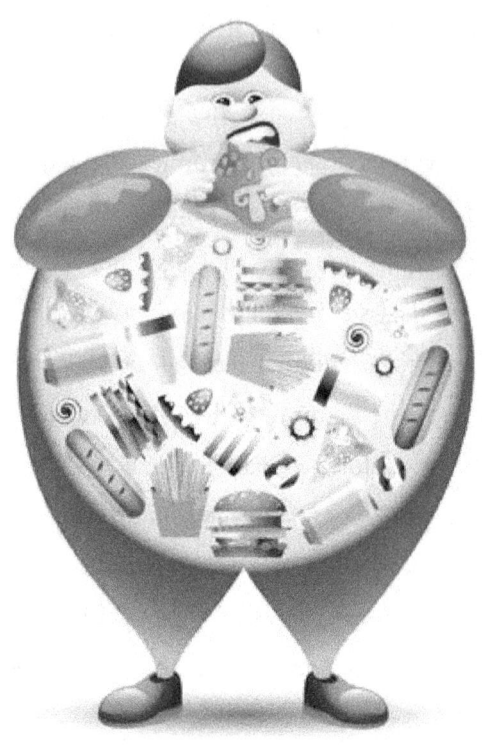

The food that a person eats contains energy in various forms like fats, carbohydrates, and proteins. These components are picked up and stored in the form of ATP. To do so, the stomach and the small intestine must break the food into hundreds of thousands of molecules which enter into the bloodstream and make their way to every cell in the human body. There they go to a small structure known as mitochondria, where the molecule goes through a number of reactions that lead to the inception of ATP. The body stores only a tiny amount of this molecule, but manufactures it quickly, as the body's requirement increase. Sometimes, while the body is still under physical stress, the demand for energy increases so the cells produce more ATP. In order to do this, they tap into the source of glucose stored in the muscles and fats stored in various places. These components then enter the bloodstream and make their way into different parts of the body via the circulatory system.

The stored glucose is known as glycogen and the fat may be broken down for the production of ATP in the following two ways:

i.   Aerobic

ii.   Anaerobic

Aerobic processes are the ones that require oxygen and produce more ATP molecules. Oxygen is their life line and they halt if the supply chain is broken. If the body works so hard it becomes impossible for it to deliver on oxygen, then the body switches to anaerobic production which has a byproduct of lactic acid. This lactic acid naturally enters into the blood and creates an imbalance. To counter this imbalance, the body increases its breathing speed so that more oxygen is taken in and the heart beats at a faster rate so the oxygen can reach the muscles.

But the anaerobic activity can't be sustained as the body can only cancel out the imbalance for a short period of time since the heart and lungs are working at full throttle. The generated lactic acid leaves a fatigued feeling and eventually the person needs to slow down. By doing so, the body gets ample supply of oxygen and once again the process of ATP production becomes aerobic. The production of lactic acid stops and the muscles start to regain their former strength.

The level of a person's fitness can be determined by the speed at which this happens. Regular exercise trains the lungs, heart, and the blood transportation mechanism, which enables them to deliver a larger quantity of oxygen to blood vessels and at a higher, swifter rate. Walking up a hill can illustrate this point.

The body is not bound to one process for the generation of ATP, but actually relies on both. Because of this there are two types of distinctions between all types of exercises:

i.   Aerobic,

ii.   Anaerobic,

If the intensity of the exercise is so high that the heart and lungs are unable to meet the demand of the muscles then the activity is anaerobic, otherwise it is aerobic.

The American College of Sports Medicine has a standard amount of time that it recommends to individuals for physical activity, i.e. 30 to 45 minutes at a frequency of 3 days in a week. Each work out should have at least 5 minutes of warm up and cool down so the body can set in and out. The American Cancer Society also recommends at least 30 minutes of physical activity that is carried out at a moderate intensity for at least 5 days per week. Children should be spending 60 minutes on medium intensity moderation exercises. Moderate exercises, like walking, will have a similar effect on the energy bill as a longer session, so choose a session that is enjoyable.

The maintenance, gain, and loss of weight are pretty much related to energy balance. Positive balance leads to an increase in weight while a negative balance leads to loss. The physical activity and caloric activity are the quantities that are balanced. Exercise is a great way to tip the scales to zero, which can help the body gain lean mass by burning more fat content than calories. Walking, or any physical activity for that sake, can burn 3 times more calories than sitting would.

It must also be known that weight loss, similar in nature to diet, can be reached by exercising alone. An exercise program that is worth a minimum of 200 minutes and focusses on moderate intensity exercises can reduce the amount of fat and general mass in body. An exercise program with less than 150 minutes training time can improve the body's cardio profile; there is an improvement in the body's overall nature as well. Exercise also improves the maintenance of the body once it loses weight, which makes it so much more superior as compared to artificial treatments.

Chapter # 3: Exercise & the Body

The cardiovascular system is responsible for transporting oxygen to the cells in the body and removing waste products from it. Moreover, it transports the necessary hormones to the different parts of the body. Moderate activities like walking do not place any excess amount of demand on the body, but when you exercise intensely, the body requires more nutrients which cause the heart to start pumping blood at a faster rate. The amount of blood put into the system has a direct impact upon the amount of oxygen it holds, which in turn, reflects the performance of muscles. Once again, the level of conditioning can dictate the working of your system. The muscles working overtime have their arteries dilated so that the increased amount of blood can easily flow. Also, the heart's increased output rate causes the blood pressure to increase, which results in the tiny arteries in the skin to expand, resulting in more blood flow. As one continues to exercise, more blood gets diverted to the skin so that a safe level of temperature is maintained.

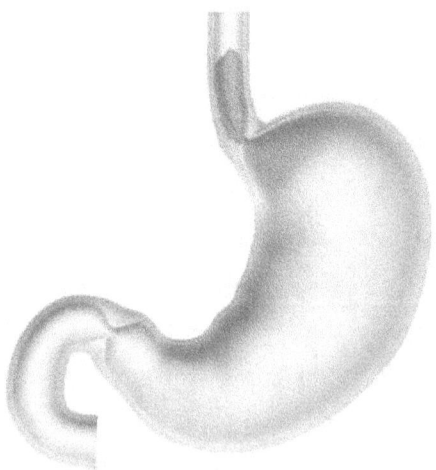

When the arteries dilate, the veins that serve the various parts of the body contract in size, and when a person rests, these veins store about 70% of the body's supply. When they contract, they make the blood available to the muscles as well as the heart, which further optimizes the distribution of blood to organs. When a person exercises regularly, his/her circulatory system adjusts itself to endure all these conditions. The body generates plasma which is a salty liquid that carries necessary components to the cells and carries away the waste products. As plasma is a part of the blood alongside the blood cells, a greater volume of blood is thus made available to the body. The blood is thinner than before which decreases the amount of resistance it faces when it circulates in different organs and parts of the body. The primary pumping units of the heart are called the ventricles which stretch so that more blood can be held. This allows for contraction with greater force, and with the passage of time the muscle located in the heart increases in size which increases its strength.

The increased need for blood containing nutrients occurs during aerobic activities, which leads to an increased number of branches of the coronary arteries that feed the heart. These arteries provide more channels for the blood to travel to the muscles of the heart, so if an artery is at risk of getting clotted, the alternate arteries take over, which keeps the flow of blood continuous. The boost in oxygen also benefits the body by warding off dangerous disturbances with respect to the heart's rhythm.

What happens when you decide to move a muscle of the body? What happens is that the brain transmits a message to the fibers in the muscles through the nerves and these fibers contract, which results in a movement. For instance, when the biceps need to be contracted, the triceps are in a relaxed state. Exercise involves all kinds of motion like walking and swimming that produces rhythmic contraction and relaxation of muscles. Moreover, this process helps the blood move through the veins and right back to where it first came from; the heart. Aerobic exercise can increase the number of fibers containing myoglobin which permits even more oxygen to store inside the muscles. Increased blood flow, alongside a greater quantity of capillaries, causes an improvement in one's endurance. Well trained muscles are therefore not just able to store more glucose, but are also able to burn more fat, directly keeping the glycogen stores saved.

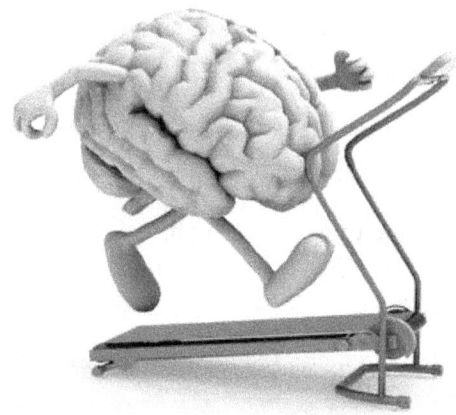

Throughout a person's life, bones are constantly building as well as dismantling. This constant process helps maintain the skeleton and frees up calcium, which is the building block of the bone. Calcium is not just vital for the bones, but it also helps a lot of other processes that go on in the body like controlling the blood pressure and heart rate. If the amount of calcium in the blood gets low then the body is forced to rely on the reservoir of calcium in the bones. When a person is young, the rate of bone formation is much faster than the rate of bone loss. But with age, the loss increases rapidly and eventually the bones become susceptible to fractures. Exercise plays a key role in slowing down this bone loss. The muscles are joined with the bones through cords called tendons, which tug the bones during all types of physical activity. The stresses that the tendons face increase the density of bones as well as their strengths. Exercises that focus on working against gravity provide the greatest benefits to the bones.

Exercise can also affect the amount of hormones released in the body. Two hormones which are key in making physical changes are released as a result of exercising. As the brain detects movement, it releases chemicals that speed up the heart, contract the blood vessels, and stimulate the release of fats as well as sugars from the body's energy reserves.

While you exercise:

- Your heart rate can hit as high as 150 beats per minute which is nearly double the amount of normal heartbeat, i.e. 80 beats per minute.

- Your skin can receive up to 80 percent of the blood flow which is quadruple the normal flow.

- The lungs pass up to 200 pints of air in and out of the body each minute, which is way too high compared to the normal flow rate, i.e. 12.

Hard-core Work Out

Chapter # 1: Introduction

Imagine that you're lying on a beach; the weather is hot and ocean air is soothing your body every time it touches you. Lying and enjoying the bright sunlight for a moment, you open your eyes and catch a glimpse of your own body, nicely toned and ripped. How did all this happen? Did it happen in hours or months? No. It happened after months of hard training which came, not from lying, but from actually doing something. So telling you that the program would be easy would be nothing more than falsehood. The book won't make such promises. Instead you should know that it will get tough, but remember, to gain something you must go through the hardships. You will have to go to a gym for this routine and will have to train under the supervision of a qualified trainer.

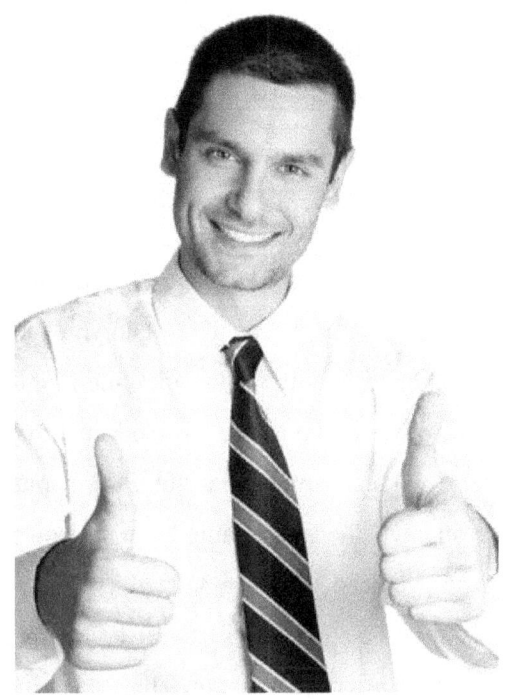

By now you must have realized that body building is an old sport; eating three meals a day whereas a normal person wants to keep on churning. But one must know that a body builder has a passion for his/her body and wants to shape it to its perfection. What this section will explain is how to lose weight by increasing one's metabolism and gaining lean mass to show off to the ladies! So read on and follow the 12 week training protocol.

What are the two main ingredients for this exercise?

1.   Aerobics

2.   Strength training

When these two join forces, they can produce immeasurable results.

Aerobics, as you might know by now, is a vital part of any weight losing program. This program includes aerobics only twice a week and only for 30 minutes, so don't worry at all. This aerobics session will have great fat cutting benefits and will have a profound effect on your metabolic rate. It is recommended that you closely monitor your weight as you exercise.

The next ingredient is weight training, which is a technique that is ignored by a lot of people who are trying to reduce fat. Did you know that strength training is very good at conditioning the muscles and if you ignore this type of training, then you would end up losing muscle rather than just fat? This is a dieter's worst enemy and can ruin his/her life. Simply put, the more amount of muscle you pack, the greater amount of fat you will burn and if you ignore lifting, then you can say good-belated-bye to your muscle. Strength training also has the added ability to raise your metabolism level and keep it that way, even after the workout. Thus, it is vital to hit the gym and the strength training routine. In this section is the backbone of the whole regimen, so it cannot be avoided in any case.

Here is the whole regimen broken down into a daily pattern:

Day	Areas to cover
Monday	Chest, triceps and shoulders
Tuesday	Cardio and abs
Wednesday	Hamstrings, calves and quads
Thursday	Abs and cardio
Friday	Biceps, forearms and back

Saturday	Rest
Sunday	Rest

Chapter # 2: Mondays

The first day, or Monday, focuses on the chest, triceps and shoulders.

The chest exercises include:

i.   **Barbell flat bench press** – this exercise needs to be performed in sets of 3 with each set in a descending order with respect to reps, i.e. 10, 8, 6. After a period of 21 days, replace this exercise with **Dumbbell Flat Bench Press** followed by reversal to the original exercise after 3 more weeks.

ii.   **Barbell incline bench press** – this exercise needs to be performed to failure, i.e. 10, 8, 6. This time you need to shift to Dumbbell incline bench press after 21 days.

iii.   **Dumbbell flys** – 1 set is to be performed containing 10 reps.

iv.   **Inclined dumbbell flys** – 1 set is to be performed that would contain 10 reps.

v.   **Dumbbell flys** – For this particular exercise, pick a very light weight and don't go to failure; keep stretching the chest for 12 reps.

The shoulder exercises include:

i.   **Seated Dumbbell presses** – Perform 3 sets to failure, i.e. 10, 8, 6.

ii.   **Standing lateral raises** – Perform 3 sets to failure, i.e. 10, 8, 6. After 21 days of seated dumbbell presses along with lateral raises, stop these exercises and replace them with upright rows for 5 sets with each set decreasing the previous one by 2 reps. After 28 days switch back to the original exercises.

The triceps exercises include:

i.   **Cable press downs** – Perform 3 sets to failure, i.e. 10, 8, 6. After 21 days of this exercise, shift to lying extensions and then shift back to the original one after 3 more weeks.

ii.   **Dumbbell kickbacks** – Perform 3 sets to failure.

The book states to perform these exercises to failure. What does this mean? This means to keep lifting until you can't lift anymore no matter how hard you try. When put in numerical form, it means that the first chosen weight should allow you to do 10 reps, the next one 8 and so on. Your lifting speed should be under control as well and you shouldn't keep throwing around weights without having any real control. Take a second to lift the weight and keep it there for a moment before lowering it with full control. It is also vital to rest in between the sets for a minute to two, as it would replenish the body's oxygen supply. It should be noted that no matter how hard you try, until or unless you break out of your comfort zone, you won't be able to gain the amount of lean mass and lose fat you wish to.

Chapter # 3: Tuesdays and Thursdays

These are cardio days and are aimed at increasing the maximum heart rate by 60 to 70 percent; any machine may be used to accomplish this task.

The abs exercises include:

i.   **Lying leg raises** – carry out at least 30 of these raises and then hold the legs for at least half a minute, about 8 inches above the ground.

ii.   **Crunches** – begin with 20 crunches and end up with 50

iii.   **Twisting crunches** – these are crunches that focus one set on each of the sides; start up with 20 or so and end up with 50.

iv.   **Crunches** – again with 20 crunches and end up with 50

Make sure to rest for about half a minute in between sets before working out again.

It must be noted that cardio is a very important segment of your exercise routine. It burns out fat at a high rate and is responsible for keeping the body on its toes. If the body gets used to working out in a similar manner, it will burn fewer calories, which means a slower metabolic rate. Therefore, a person must avoid performing the same exercise every day.

- For the first cardio week, use the elliptical cross trainer exercise machine.

- For the second week use a stationary bike.

- For the third week use a stair master.

- For the fourth week start over from the top.

The point of this routine is simple, if you keep on changing the workout pattern the body will not get used to it and you will have an ever increasing metabolism rate.

Chapter # 4: Wednesdays

These are leg days and are probably the one that come across the most frightening.

The hamstrings and quads exercises include:

i.   **Leg presses** – perform three sets of leg presses or squats to failure.

ii.   **Leg extensions** – At first perform three sets of the exercise to exhaustion, but after 21 days replace this exercise with sissy squats. Perform three sets of these exercises as well, with 10 reps. When using these exercises, stretch for at least 3 minutes; do the basic thighs stretch as well as the groin stretch.

iii.   **Lying leg curls** – Perform 3 sets of this exercise till failure. After 21 days replace this exercise with standing leg curls; perform 3 sets to failure. After 3 more weeks switch back and once again stretch out using the basic hamstring stretch.

The calf exercises include:

i.   **Seated calf raises** – Perform five sets of seated calf raises for the first 21 days. After 21 days, replace this exercise with standing calf raises. After another 21 days, replace the exercise back to seated calf raises.

Your lifting speed throughout the exercises should be under control and you shouldn't be throwing stuff around. Take some time to lift the object. Similarly, the exercise to failure means to work out until you can't lift anymore and to pick a weight in the range which allows you to go within the prescribed range.

It is also vital to rest in between sets to replenish your bodily supplies. Resting for two to three minutes in between different muscle exercises is recommended.

Chapter # 5: Fridays

This is the last day of the week you have to work out.

The hamstrings and quads exercises include:

i.   **Machine pull downs (lateral)** – Perform these exercises in sets of 5 to failure. After a period of 21 days, switch to the close gripped version of pull downs and after another 21 days switch to wide grip pull downs. If you want to, you may execute wide grip chin ups.

ii.   **Dumbbell rows** – perform three sets of 10, 8, and 6 to failure and after 21 days replace the exercise with seated cable rows.

iii.   **Bent dumbbell laterals** – perform 3 sets of equal reps for 21 days before switching to seated version; switch back to the original after 3 more weeks.

The biceps exercises include:

i.   **Standing barbell curls** – Use curl or normal bars to perform 3 sets of this exercise; the procedure is the same and the exercise is to be performed till failure. Replace this exercise with seated dumbbell curls after 21 days.

ii.   **Concentration curls** – Perform 3 sets of this exercise to failure; the sets are the same as the previous exercise. After 21 days replace it with the alternate dumbbell curls.

The forearms exercises include:

i.   **Reverse barbell curls** – Perform three sets of this exercise to failure; the number of sets is the same, i.e. 10, 8, 6.

ii.   **Barbell wrist curls** – perform three sets of this exercise to failure; the number of sets is the same.

These exercises also have the same rules as the previous ones. When the book states to do the exercise to failure, you must pay special attention at picking up the weight. Moreover, the lifting speed must also be checked; take 1 to 1.5 seconds to lift a weight and take 2 to lower it down.

Rest for a minute to 1.5 minutes in between sets, and rest for 3 minutes in between different groups. This is a great workout for strengthening as well conditioning the back and for the biceps. You will probably burn more calories than any other day of the week.

Chapter # 6: Alternate

It must be known that each and every individual has a personalized and customized working out plan, which must be respected. Some individuals work out at different times than others, so here are two alternate splits which you can follow:

1.　　**Split # 1:**

Monday – Shoulders, chest, and triceps

Tuesday – Abs and cardio

Wednesday – Hamstrings, calves plus quads

Thursday – Abs and cardio

Friday – Back, biceps, and forearms

Saturday and Sunday - off

Split # 2:

Monday – Shoulders, chest and triceps

Tuesday – Abs and cardio

Wednesday – Back, biceps, and forearms

Thursday – Abs and cardio

Friday – Hamstrings, quads, and calves

Saturday and Sunday - off

I say it again, this is not an easy workout, but if you do it with the goal of cutting fat then you will definitely succeed. The key is to keep asking yourself the question about what you truly want; a ripped body or one with diseases. You must not forget that to get something you must be willing to work for it, because there is no easy way to success.

Conclusion

Exercise is vital for proper health, as well as weight loss. If you don't engage yourself in some kind of physical activity, then you'll end up contracting a lot of problems; one of which would be gaining weight. Obesity is becoming an uncontrollable health condition which is affecting millions around the world. Medical companies are putting forward products which provide only short term relief, but in the long term fail a person. The only true way to conquer this condition is through proper exercise which is the topic of this book. All of the relevant information has been given in the book so you can easily get those extra pounds off you. Stay motivated and keep following the training plan to succeed.

Best of luck!

References

https://www.fotolia.com/id/39676947

https://www.fotolia.com/id/40822406

https://www.fotolia.com/id/42606253

https://www.fotolia.com/id/45156048

https://www.fotolia.com/id/51102457

https://www.fotolia.com/id/18623490

Author Bio

Muhammad Usman is a distinguished medical graduate of Allama Iqbal medical college (AIMC). He is a professional writer who has been in the field for more than 4 years. During this time he has produced 10,000+ articles, blogs and eBooks on various niches related to diseases, health, fitness, nutrition and well-being. He is a regular contributor to several journals related to medicine and surgery. He is the editor of several journals and newspapers.

Check out some of the other JD-Biz Publishing books

Gardening Series on Amazon

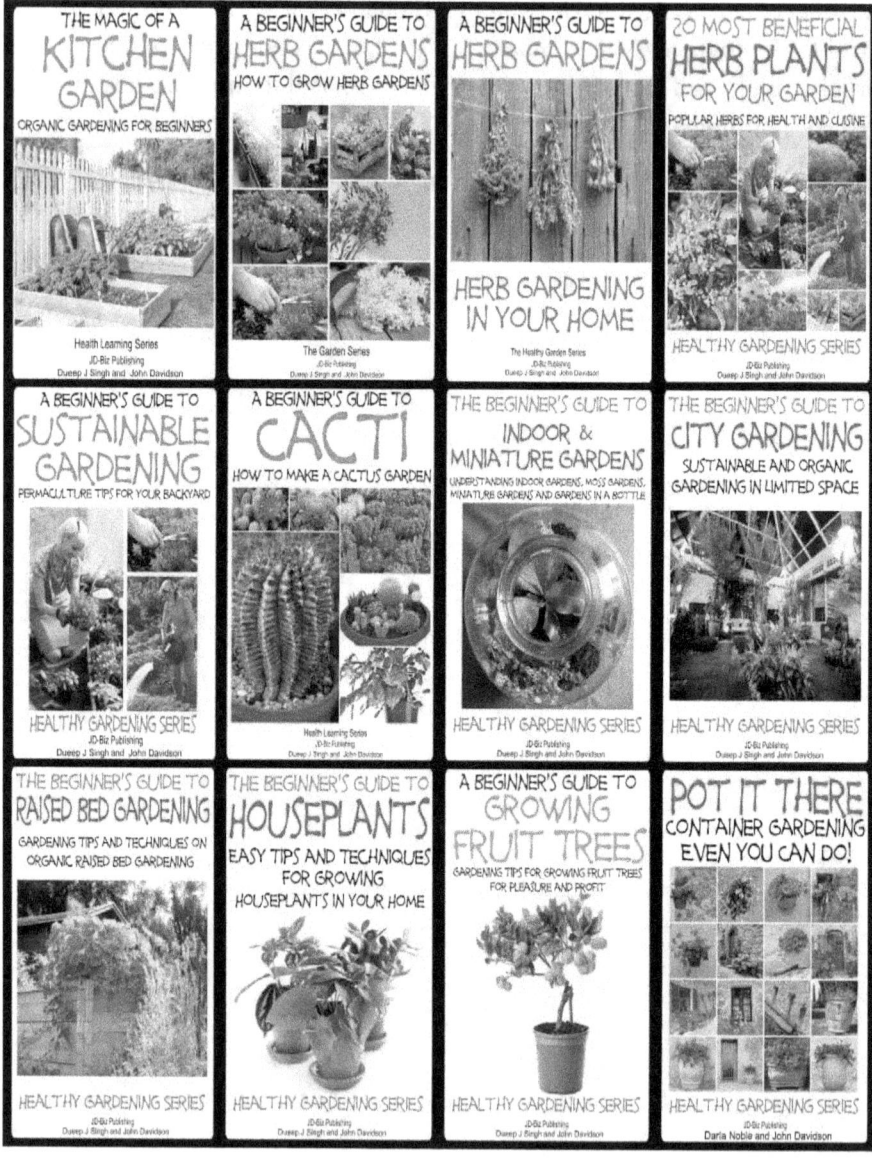

Health Learning Series

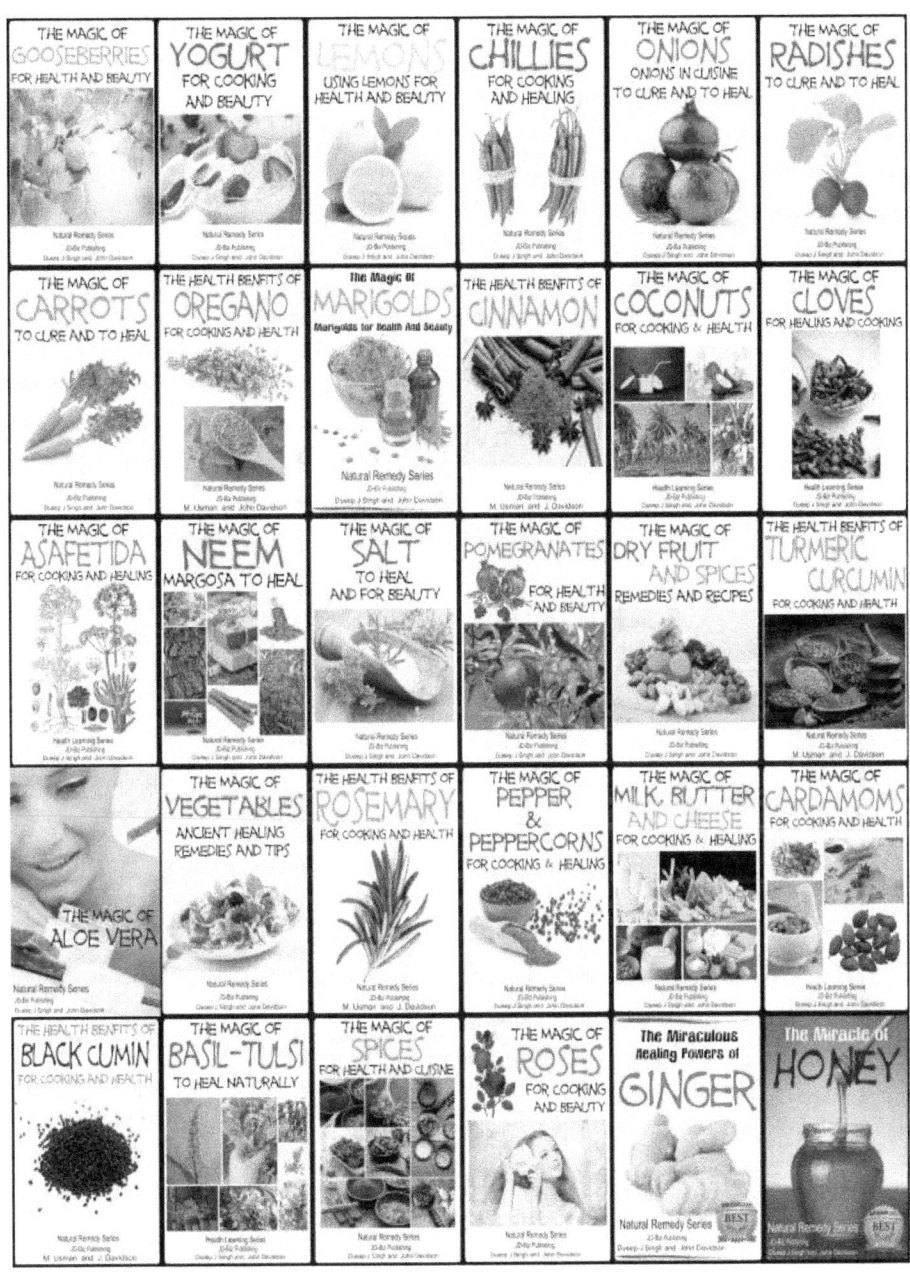

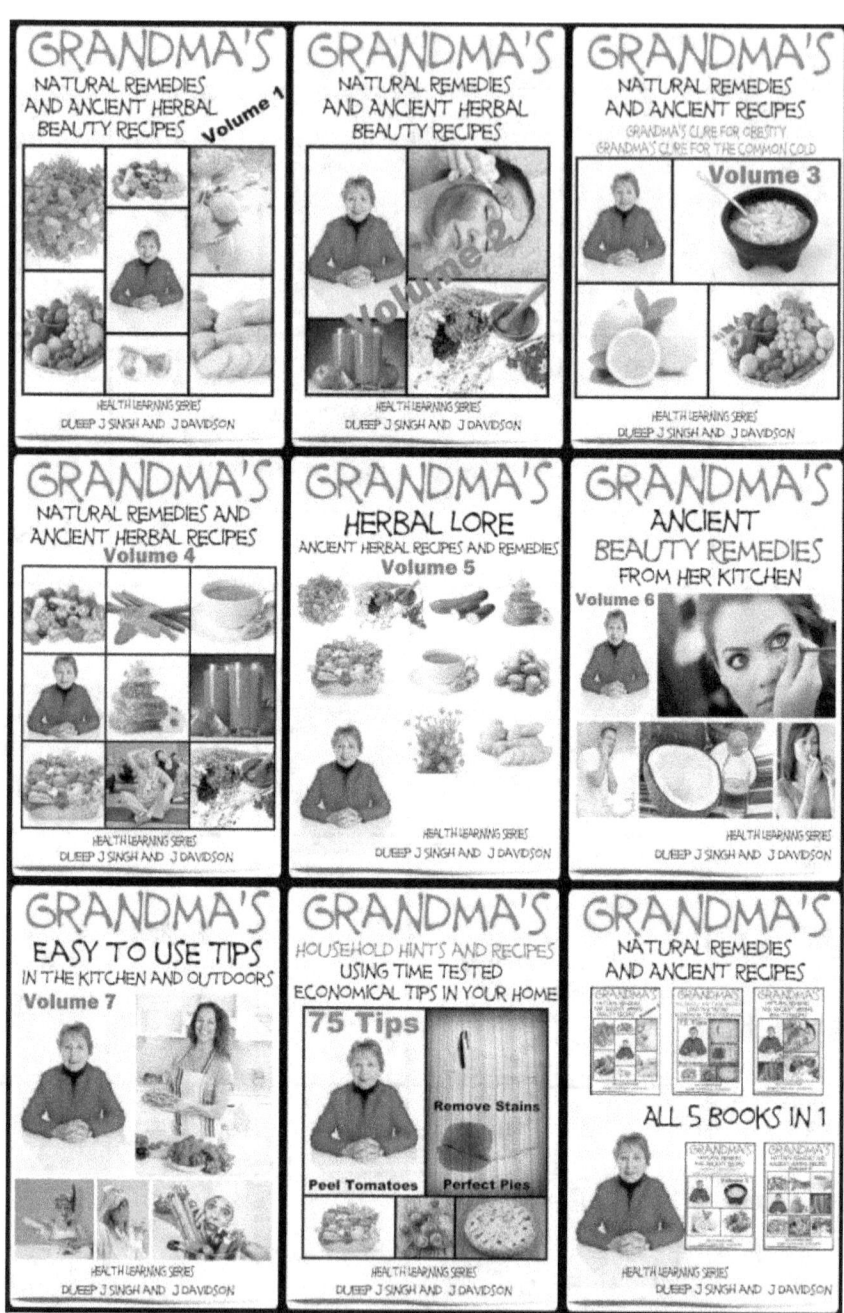

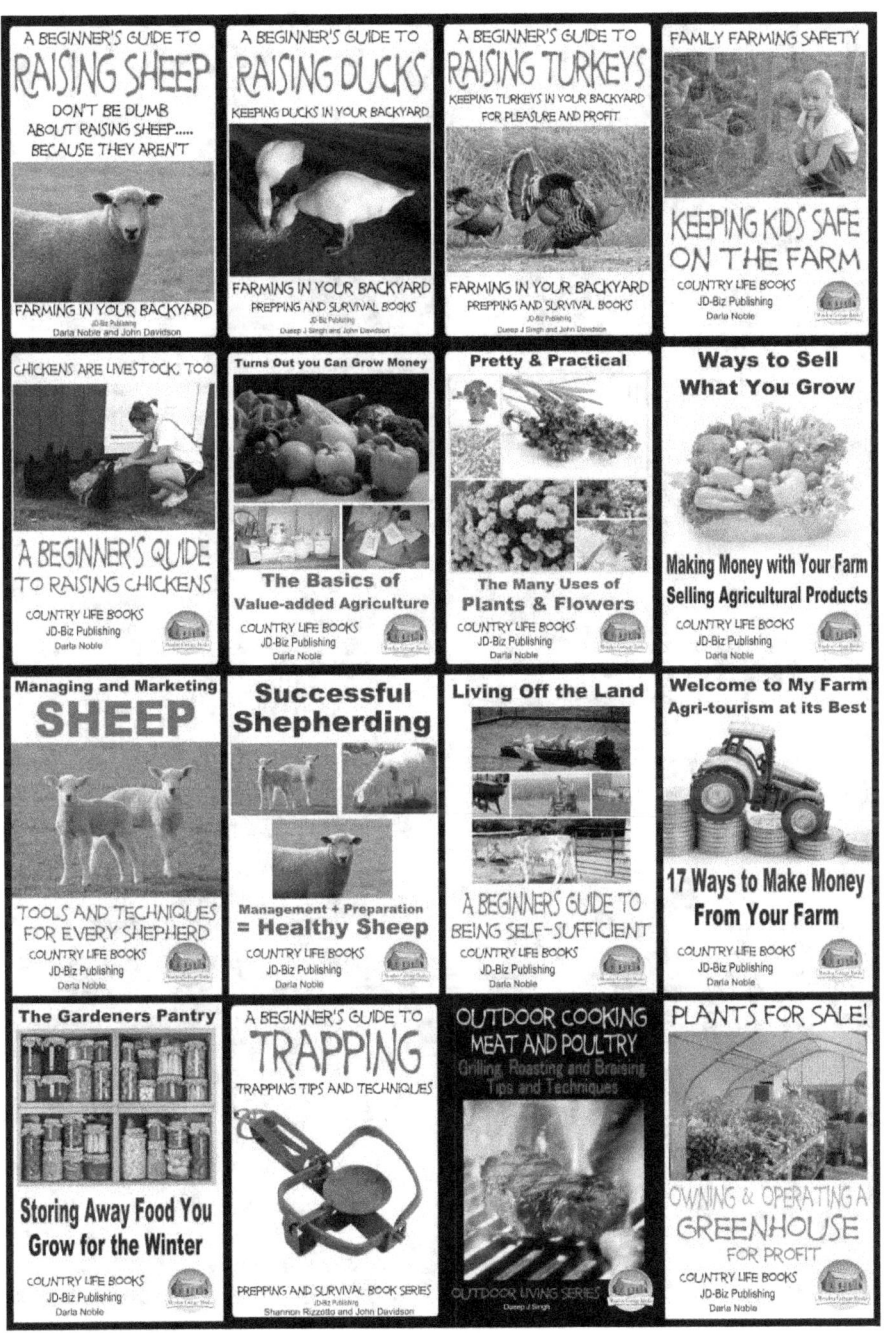

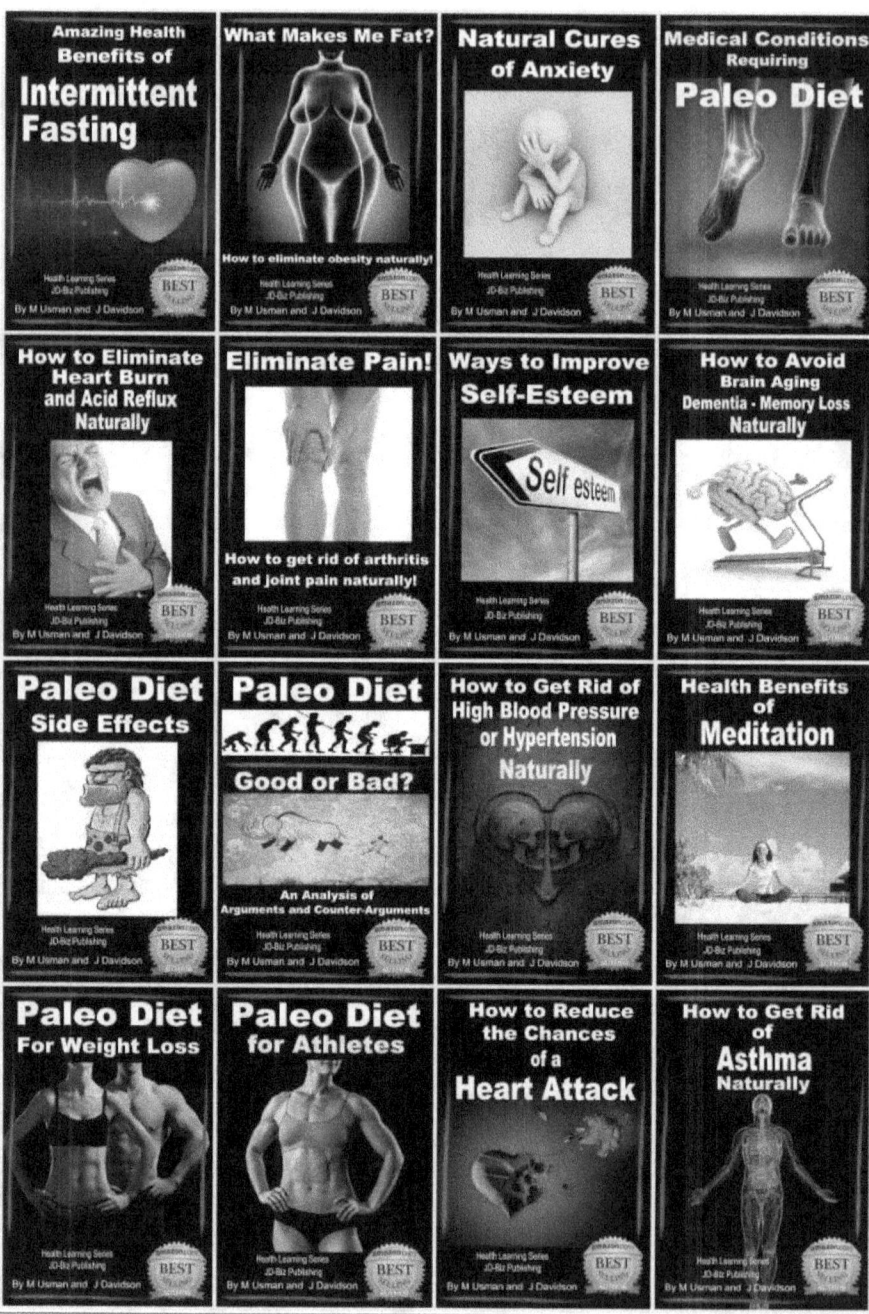

<u>Amazing Animal Book Series</u>

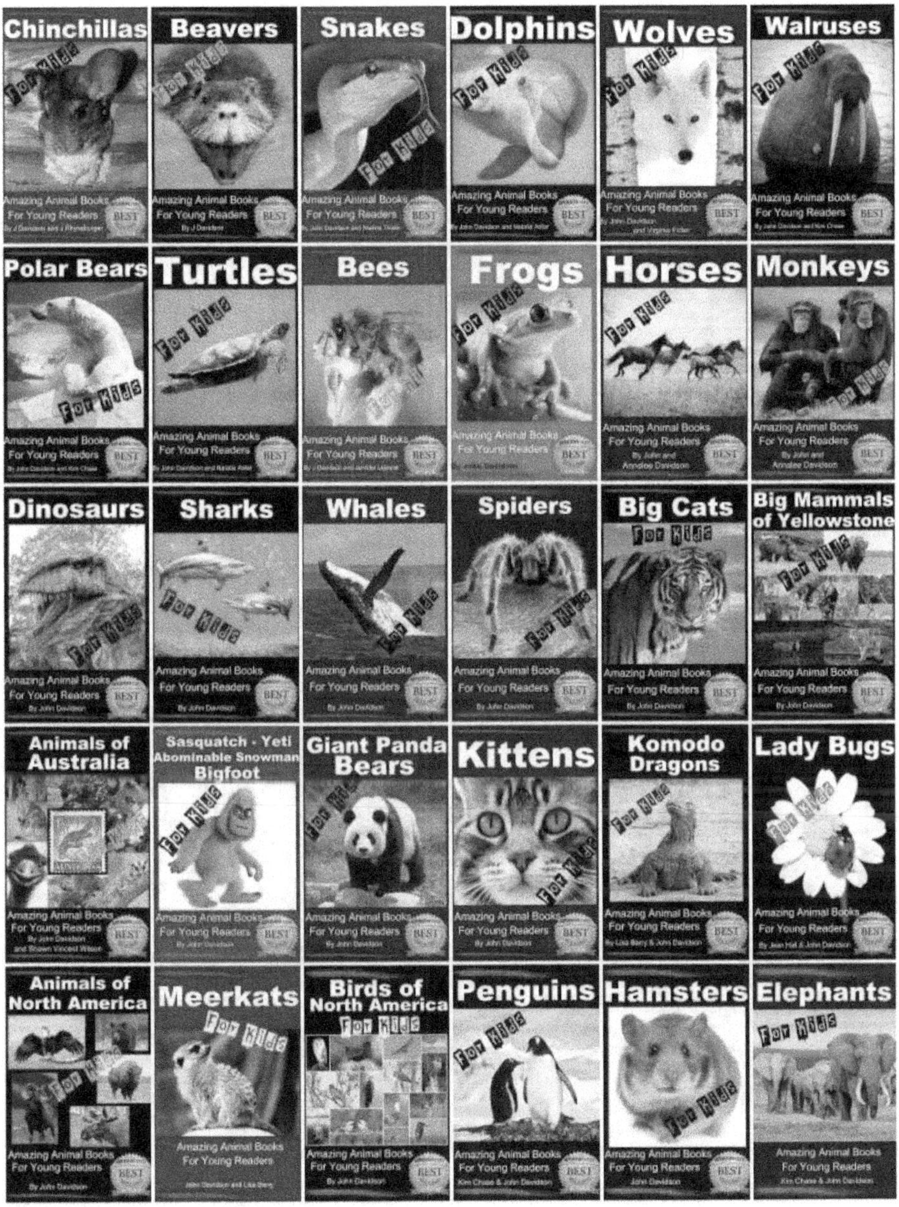

Learn To Draw Series

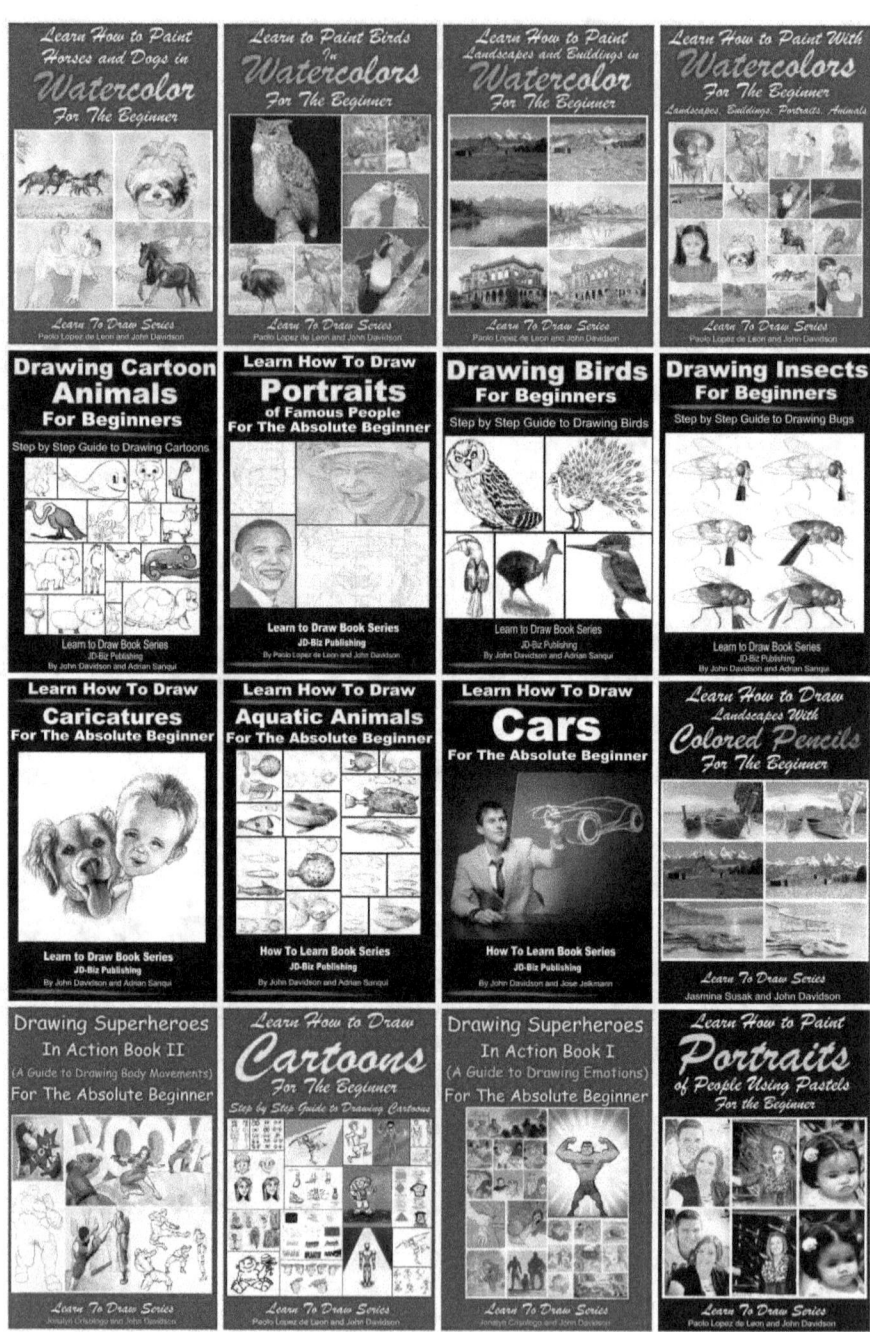

How to Build and Plan Books

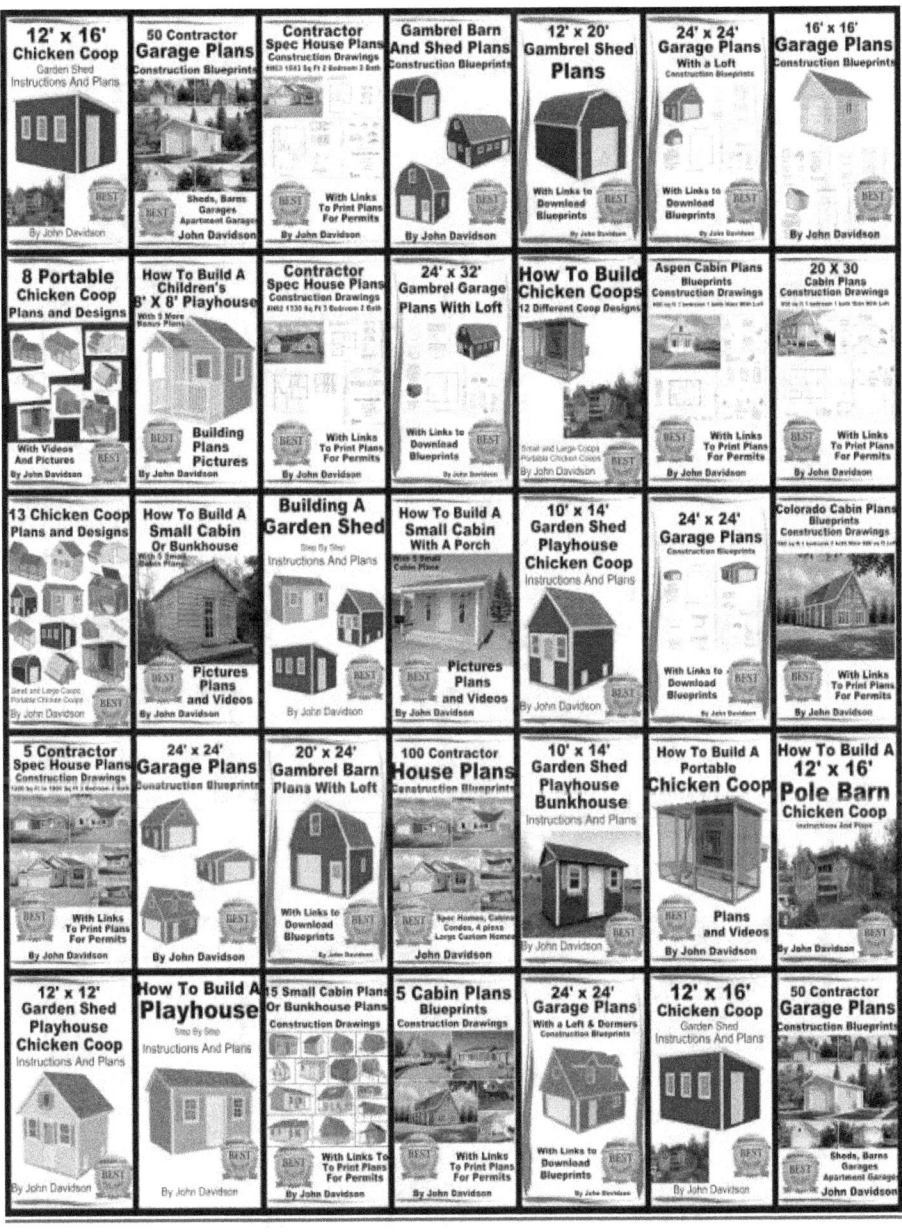

Entrepreneur Book Series

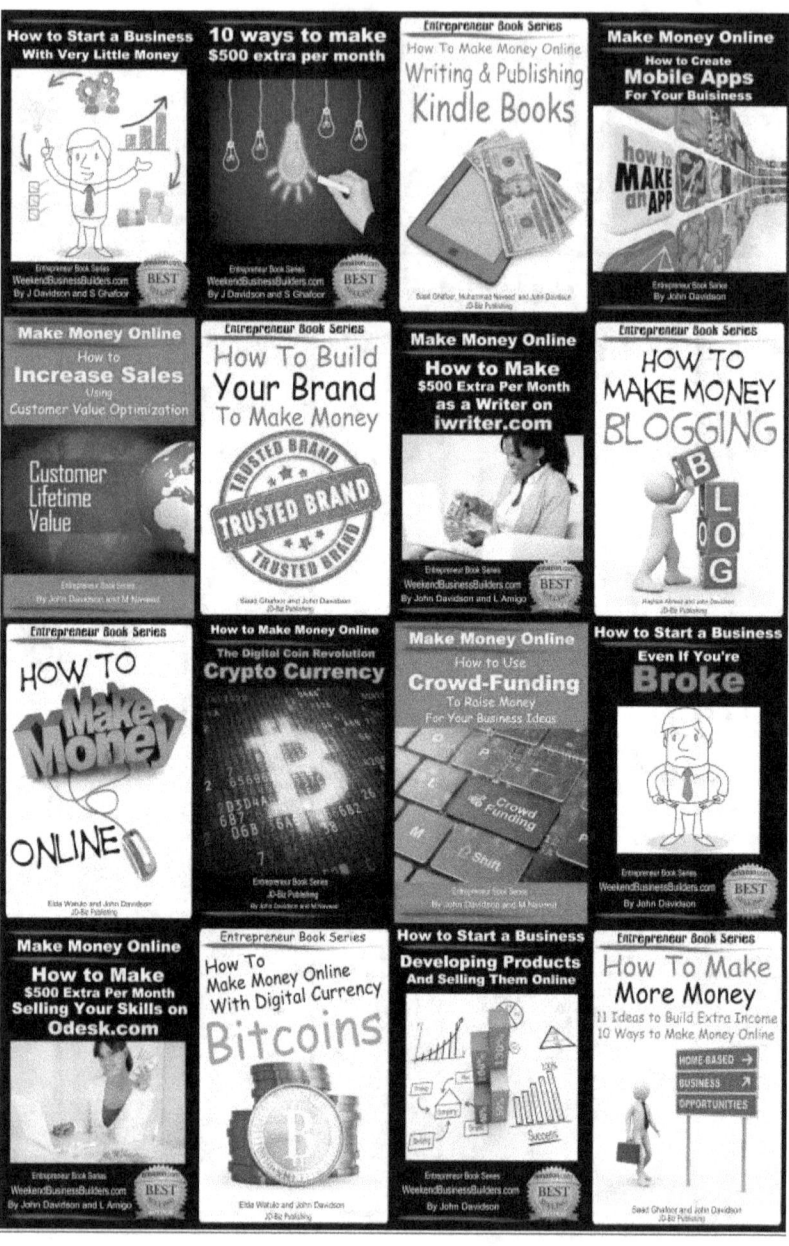

Our books are available at

1. Amazon.com

2. Barnes and Noble

3. Itunes

4. Kobo

5. Smashwords

6. Google Play Books

Publisher

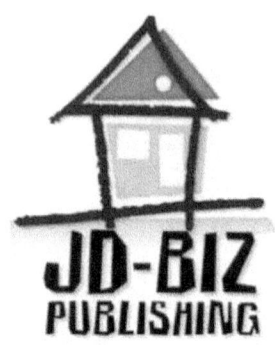

JD-Biz Corp

P O Box 374

Mendon, Utah 84325

http://www.jd-biz.com/

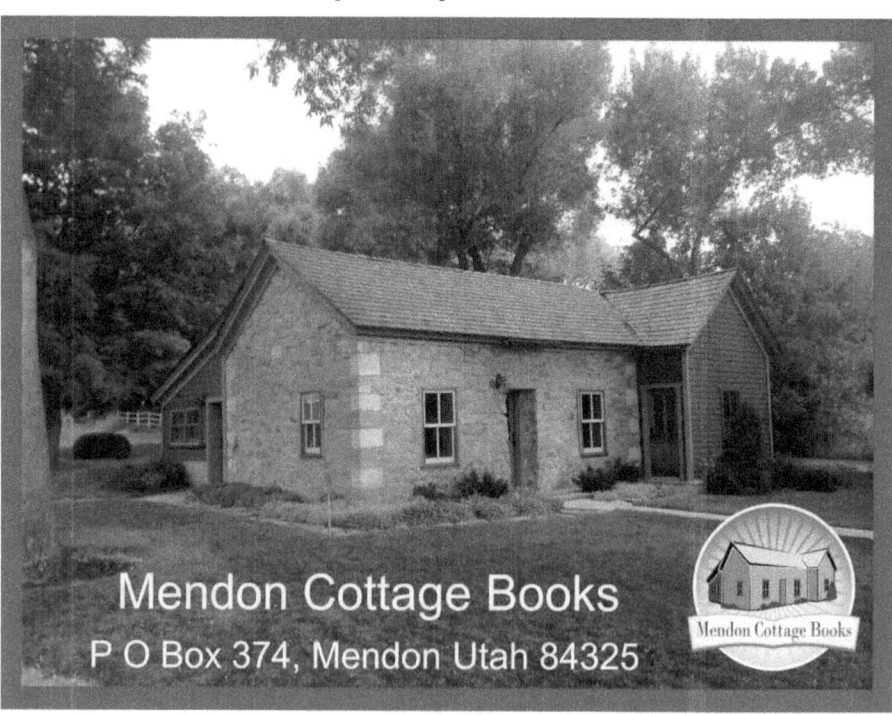